This publication is intended to provide educational information for the reader on the covered subjects. It is not intended to take the place of personalized medical counseling, diagnosis, and treatment from a trained healthcare professional.

ISBN 978-1-998740-19-2 (Paperback)
ISBN 978-1-998740-20-8 (eBook)

Printed and bound in USA
Published by Loons Press

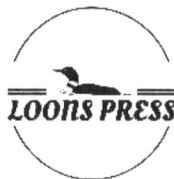

I0106281

LOONS PRESS

# Table Of Contents

| | |
|---|---|
| **Chapter 1** | **6** |
| **Understanding Health and Happiness** | **6** |
| The Connection Between Body and Mind | 6 |
| Defining Health and Happiness | 9 |
| The Importance of Balance | 11 |
| **Chapter 2** | **15** |
| **Nutrition for a Healthy Body** | **15** |
| Understanding Nutrients | 15 |
| Building a Balanced Diet | 18 |
| Meal Planning and Preparation | 21 |
| **Chapter 3** | **25** |
| **Physical Activity and Fitness** | **25** |
| The Benefits of Regular Exercise | 25 |
| Finding the Right Exercise for You | 28 |
| Creating a Sustainable Fitness Routine | 30 |
| **Chapter 4** | **35** |

**Mental Wellness and Mindfulness** 35

The Role of Mental Health in Overall Wellbeing 35

Introduction to Mindfulness Practices 38

Techniques for Reducing Stress 41

**Chapter 5** 45

**Building Healthy Relationships** 45

The Impact of Relationships on Health 45

Effective Communication Skills 48

Setting Boundaries for Healthy Interactions 50

**Chapter 6** 54

**Sleep and Recovery** 54

The Importance of Sleep for Health 54

Sleep Hygiene Practices 57

Understanding Recovery and Rest 60

**Chapter 7** 64

**Emotional Intelligence and Resilience** 64

What is Emotional Intelligence? 64

Developing Resilience 67

Coping Strategies for Life Challenges 70

**Chapter 8** **75**

**Creating a Healthy Environment** **75**

The Influence of Your Surroundings 75

Decluttering and Organizing for Peace 78

Incorporating Nature into Daily Life 81

**Chapter 9** **86**

**Setting Goals for Health and Happiness** **86**

The Importance of Goal Setting 86

SMART Goals for Wellness 89

Tracking Progress and Adjusting Goals 92

**Chapter 10** **96**

**Maintaining Balance in Daily Life** **96**

Time Management for Health 96

Finding Joy in Daily Activities 99

Strategies for Long-term Balance 101

**Author Notes & Acknowledgments** **105**

**Author Bio** **107**

# How To Be Healthy and Happy

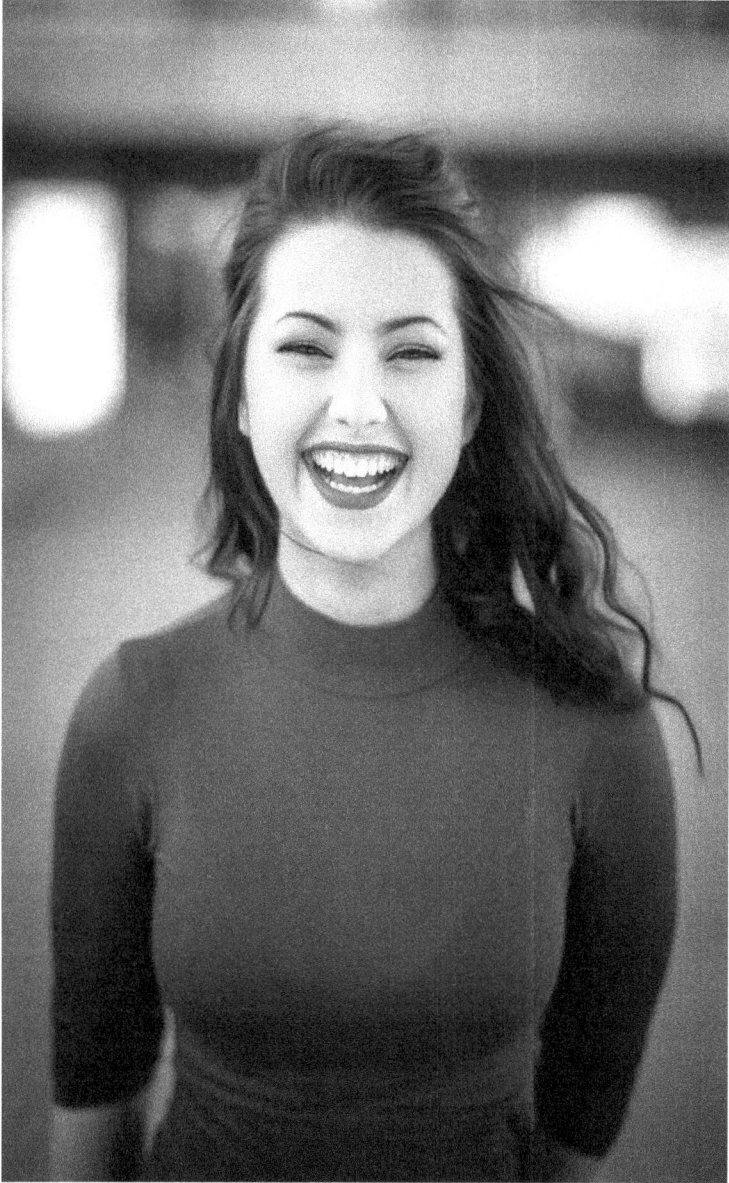

# Chapter 1

# Understanding Health and Happiness

## The Connection Between Body and Mind

The connection between body and mind is a fundamental aspect of overall health and happiness. This intricate relationship highlights how mental states can influence physical health and vice versa. When individuals experience stress or anxiety, for instance, it can manifest in physical symptoms such as headaches, digestive issues, or fatigue.

Conversely, engaging in physical activity can lead to improved mood and cognitive function, illustrating the bidirectional nature of this connection. Understanding and nurturing this relationship is essential for achieving a balanced and fulfilling life.

Research has consistently shown that physical health directly impacts mental well-being. Regular exercise releases endorphins, often referred to as "feel-good" hormones, which can alleviate symptoms of depression and anxiety. Furthermore, physical activity promotes better sleep patterns, which are crucial for cognitive function and emotional regulation. By incorporating regular exercise into daily routines, individuals can not only enhance their physical fitness but also cultivate a more positive mental state, fostering a sense of accomplishment and boosting self-esteem.

On the other hand, mental health plays a vital role in physical well-being. Stress management techniques such as mindfulness, meditation, and deep breathing can lower cortisol levels, reducing the risk of chronic illnesses associated with prolonged stress. Engaging in activities that promote mental clarity and emotional resilience can lead to healthier lifestyle choices, such as balanced nutrition and consistent exercise. When individuals prioritize mental health, they often find themselves more motivated to care for their bodies, creating a positive feedback loop that enhances both mind and body.

Nutrition is another critical element in the mind-body connection. The brain requires specific nutrients to function optimally, and a well-balanced diet can significantly affect mood and cognitive abilities. Foods rich in omega-3 fatty acids, antioxidants, and vitamins can bolster mental health, while a diet high in processed sugars and unhealthy fats may contribute to mood swings and cognitive decline.

By adopting a diet that nourishes both the body and mind, individuals can enhance their overall well-being and cultivate a more positive outlook on life.

Ultimately, maintaining a harmonious connection between body and mind is essential for achieving lasting health and happiness. Individuals are encouraged to adopt holistic approaches that emphasize the interdependence of physical and mental health. This may include integrating regular exercise, mindful eating, stress-reduction techniques, and self-care practices into daily life. By prioritizing both aspects, individuals can create a balanced lifestyle that fosters resilience, joy, and overall fulfillment, leading to a healthier and happier existence.

# Defining Health and Happiness

Health and happiness are often viewed as interconnected concepts, yet defining them requires a nuanced understanding. Health typically encompasses physical, mental, and emotional well-being. It is more than the absence of illness; it involves maintaining a balanced lifestyle that supports vitality and resilience. Physical health can be measured through various indicators such as fitness levels, nutrition, and the absence of disease. However, mental and emotional health are equally vital, as they influence how we perceive and interact with the world around us.

Happiness, on the other hand, is a more subjective experience. It can be defined as a state of well-being characterized by emotions ranging from contentment to intense joy. While some people find happiness in achieving personal goals, others may derive joy from relationships, experiences, or a sense of purpose. Happiness is influenced by individual perceptions and societal standards, making it a complex and often elusive state. Understanding what brings happiness to oneself is a crucial step in the journey toward overall well-being.

The relationship between health and happiness is reciprocal. Good health can lead to greater happiness, as physical well-being often provides the energy and motivation needed to pursue activities that bring joy. Conversely, happiness can enhance health by reducing stress, improving immune function, and encouraging healthier lifestyle choices. When individuals are happy, they are more likely to engage in regular exercise, maintain a nutritious diet, and practice self-care, all of which contribute to better health outcomes.

Achieving a balance between health and happiness requires a holistic approach. This involves not only tending to physical needs through diet and exercise but also nurturing mental and emotional health. Mindfulness practices, such as meditation and yoga, can help individuals cultivate a positive mindset and manage stress.

Additionally, fostering strong social connections and engaging in meaningful activities are essential components in enhancing both happiness and health. Recognizing that these elements are interdependent can empower individuals to make choices that support their overall well-being.

Ultimately, defining health and happiness is a personal journey that varies from one individual to another. Each person's values, experiences, and circumstances play a significant role in shaping their understanding of what it means to be healthy and happy. By exploring these definitions and their interplay, individuals can develop a roadmap that guides them toward a more balanced and fulfilling life. Embracing the journey of self-discovery in pursuit of health and happiness fosters resilience and equips individuals with the tools to navigate the challenges of life with grace and positivity.

## The Importance of Balance

The concept of balance is fundamental to achieving a healthy and happy life. It encompasses various aspects, including physical health, mental well-being, emotional stability, and social connections. Striking a balance among these areas is crucial for overall wellness. When individuals prioritize one area at the expense of others, they may experience stress, burnout, or dissatisfaction. Understanding the importance of balance helps individuals create a harmonious lifestyle that nurtures all facets of their being.

Physical health is often the first area people think of when considering balance. Regular exercise, a nutritious diet, and sufficient sleep are essential components of a healthy body. However, achieving balance means not only focusing on these elements but also recognizing the role of rest and recovery. Overtraining or restrictive dieting can lead to physical exhaustion and negative mental health outcomes. Thus, incorporating relaxation techniques, such as meditation or yoga, can provide a counterpoint to the demands of physical fitness, allowing the body to recover and thrive.

Mental health is equally important and closely tied to physical well-being. A balanced approach to mental health includes managing stress, cultivating a positive mindset, and seeking support when necessary. Engaging in activities that promote mental stimulation, such as reading or learning new skills, can enhance cognitive function and overall happiness. On the other hand, neglecting mental health can lead to anxiety and depression, which may further impact physical health. Therefore, prioritizing mental wellness through mindfulness and self-care practices is essential for maintaining a balanced life.

Emotional balance is another key component of well-being. It involves recognizing and managing emotions rather than suppressing them. Emotional intelligence allows individuals to navigate their feelings effectively and build healthier relationships with others. Establishing a support network of friends and family can provide emotional sustenance, helping individuals cope with life's challenges.

Furthermore, engaging in activities that bring joy and fulfillment fosters emotional balance, contributing to a more satisfying and happy life.

Finally, social connections play a vital role in achieving balance. Humans are inherently social beings, and meaningful relationships contribute significantly to happiness and health. Striking a balance between time spent alone and time spent with others is crucial. While solitude can promote self-reflection and rejuvenation, social interactions provide support and a sense of belonging. By nurturing relationships and fostering a sense of community, individuals can create a balanced life that enhances both their emotional and physical health, ultimately leading to a happier existence.

# How To Be Healthy and Happy

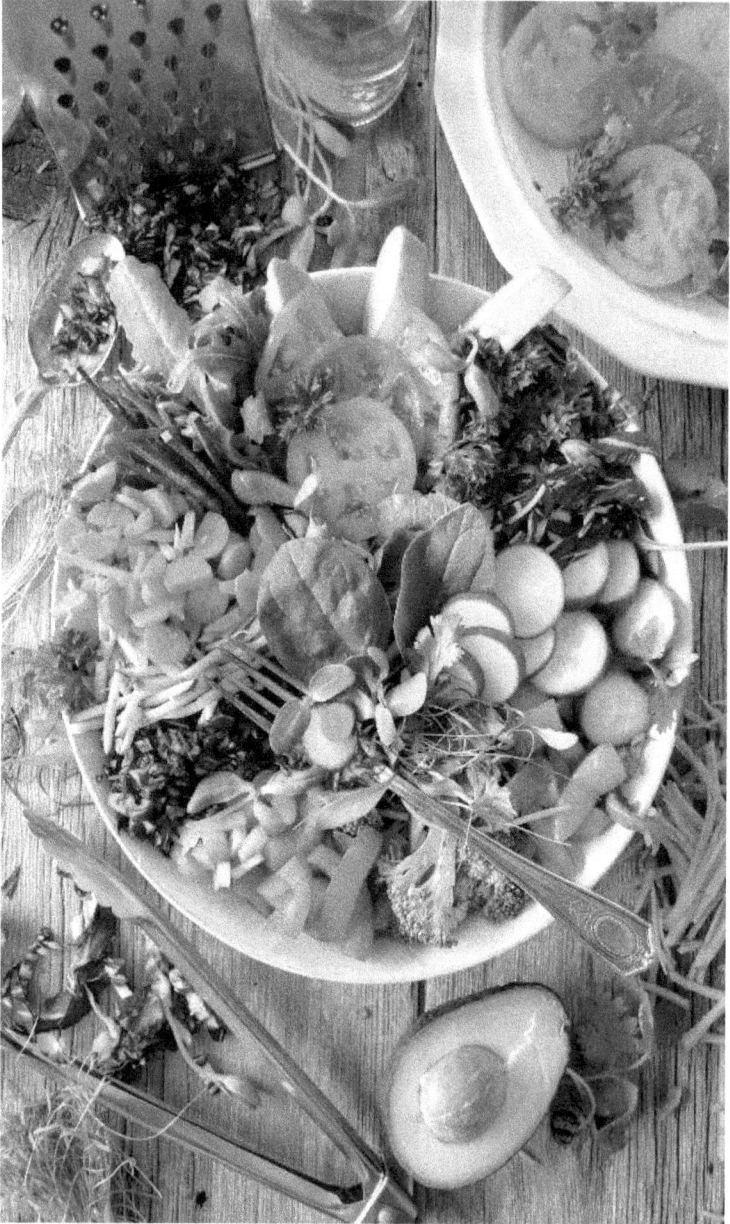

Finding Balance for Body and Mind

# Chapter 2

# Nutrition for a Healthy Body

## Understanding Nutrients

Nutrients are the building blocks of a healthy diet and play a critical role in maintaining overall well-being. They are substances that the body needs to function optimally, to grow, and to repair itself.

Understanding the different types of nutrients is essential for anyone looking to improve their health and happiness. Nutrients can be categorized into macronutrients and micronutrients, each serving distinct functions that contribute to our physical and mental health.

Macronutrients include carbohydrates, proteins, and fats, which are required in larger quantities. Carbohydrates are the body's primary source of energy, fueling everything from daily activities to complex bodily functions.

When consumed, carbohydrates are broken down into glucose, which is vital for brain function and energy. Proteins, on the other hand, are crucial for building and repairing tissues, making enzymes, and supporting immune function. Sources of protein include meat, fish, dairy, legumes, and nuts.

Fats, although often misunderstood, are essential for hormone production, nutrient absorption, and providing a concentrated source of energy. Healthy fats, such as those found in avocados, olive oil, and fish, should be prioritized over trans fats and saturated fats.

Micronutrients, which include vitamins and minerals, are required in smaller amounts but are equally important for our health. Vitamins, such as A, C, D, E, and the B-complex vitamins, play various roles in metabolism, immune function, and overall cellular health. For instance, vitamin C is vital for collagen production and immune support, while vitamin D is essential for bone health and mood regulation.

Minerals, including calcium, iron, magnesium, and potassium, are involved in numerous biochemical processes, from bone strength to energy production. A diverse diet rich in fruits, vegetables, whole grains, and lean proteins can help ensure that individuals receive a wide array of these essential nutrients.

The balance between macronutrients and micronutrients is key to achieving and maintaining a healthy lifestyle. Consuming a diet that is overly skewed toward one macronutrient can lead to deficiencies in others, potentially resulting in health issues.

For example, a diet high in carbohydrates but low in protein may hinder muscle repair and growth. Similarly, neglecting micronutrients can lead to deficiencies that impact mental health, such as low energy levels and mood swings. Monitoring one's nutrient intake can be a straightforward way to ensure that all bodily systems function effectively and harmoniously.

Ultimately, understanding nutrients empowers individuals to make informed dietary choices that promote both physical health and mental well-being. A well-rounded diet that includes a variety of foods not only satisfies hunger but also nourishes the body and mind. By prioritizing nutrient-dense foods and being mindful of dietary balance, people can enhance their overall quality of life, fostering a state of health and happiness that resonates through every aspect of their daily existence.

## Building a Balanced Diet

A balanced diet is essential for maintaining both physical health and emotional well-being. It involves consuming a variety of foods in the right proportions to provide the body with the necessary nutrients it needs to function optimally.

A well-rounded diet should include fruits, vegetables, whole grains, lean proteins, and healthy fats. Each food group contributes unique vitamins, minerals, and other nutrients that support bodily functions, making it crucial to incorporate a wide range of foods into daily meals.

Fruits and vegetables are foundational elements of a balanced diet. They are rich in vitamins, minerals, antioxidants, and dietary fiber, all of which play a significant role in promoting health. Aim to fill half your plate with these colorful foods at every meal.

Seasonal produce not only enhances flavor but also ensures that you are getting a variety of nutrients. Fresh, frozen, or canned options can all contribute to your intake, but it is best to choose those without added sugars or sodium when possible.

Whole grains are another critical component. Unlike refined grains, whole grains retain their bran and germ, which means they provide more fiber and nutrients. Incorporating sources such as brown rice, quinoa, whole wheat bread, and oats can help regulate blood sugar levels, improve digestion, and promote heart health.

It is advisable to make at least half of your grain choices whole grains to maximize health benefits and maintain balanced energy levels throughout the day.

Lean proteins are vital for muscle repair, immune function, and overall bodily maintenance. Sources such as poultry, fish, beans, legumes, and low-fat dairy provide essential amino acids without the added saturated fats found in some red meats. Including a variety of protein sources in your diet can help you meet your nutritional needs while keeping meals interesting.

It's also beneficial to consider plant-based proteins, which can contribute to heart health and reduce the risk of chronic diseases.

Finally, healthy fats should not be overlooked. Fats are essential for absorbing certain vitamins and providing energy. Sources like avocados, nuts, seeds, and olive oil offer heart-healthy fats that support brain function and overall health. It is important to limit saturated and trans fats, typically found in processed foods, to maintain a balanced diet.

By being mindful of the types and amounts of fats consumed, individuals can support their physical health and emotional well-being, ultimately contributing to a happier, healthier life.

## Meal Planning and Preparation

Meal planning and preparation are critical components of maintaining a healthy and balanced lifestyle. By taking the time to plan meals in advance, individuals can ensure they are making mindful choices that align with their health goals. This proactive approach helps eliminate the stress of last-minute decisions, which often lead to unhealthy eating habits. When meals are planned, it becomes easier to incorporate a variety of nutrients and food groups, contributing to overall well-being.

To begin effective meal planning, it is essential to assess personal dietary needs and preferences. Each individual has unique health goals, whether it be weight management, muscle gain, or simply improving overall nutrition. By understanding these goals, one can select recipes that cater to specific dietary requirements, such as low-carb, high-protein, or plant-based options.

Additionally, considering food preferences and allergies is crucial in creating a sustainable meal plan that one can stick to in the long run.

Once dietary needs are established, creating a weekly meal schedule can streamline the cooking process. This involves selecting a few recipes for breakfast, lunch, and dinner, along with healthy snacks. It is helpful to choose dishes that can be made in bulk or have overlapping ingredients, reducing waste and saving time. A well-structured meal plan not only promotes healthy eating but also encourages variety, which is important for receiving a broad spectrum of nutrients.

Preparation is equally important as planning. Setting aside time each week for meal prep can significantly enhance the likelihood of adhering to the meal plan. This can include tasks such as chopping vegetables, marinating proteins, or cooking grains in advance.

By preparing components ahead of time, individuals can easily assemble meals during busy weekdays, making healthy choices more accessible. Batch cooking and storing meals in portioned containers can also support portion control and reduce the temptation to opt for convenience foods.

Incorporating meal planning and preparation into daily life fosters a sense of control over one's diet and promotes healthier choices. It cultivates mindfulness around food, encouraging individuals to be more aware of what they consume. As a result, not only does meal planning contribute to physical health, but it also enhances mental well-being by reducing the stress associated with food decisions. By making meal planning a regular practice, individuals can find balance and satisfaction in their journey toward health and happiness.

# How To Be Healthy and Happy

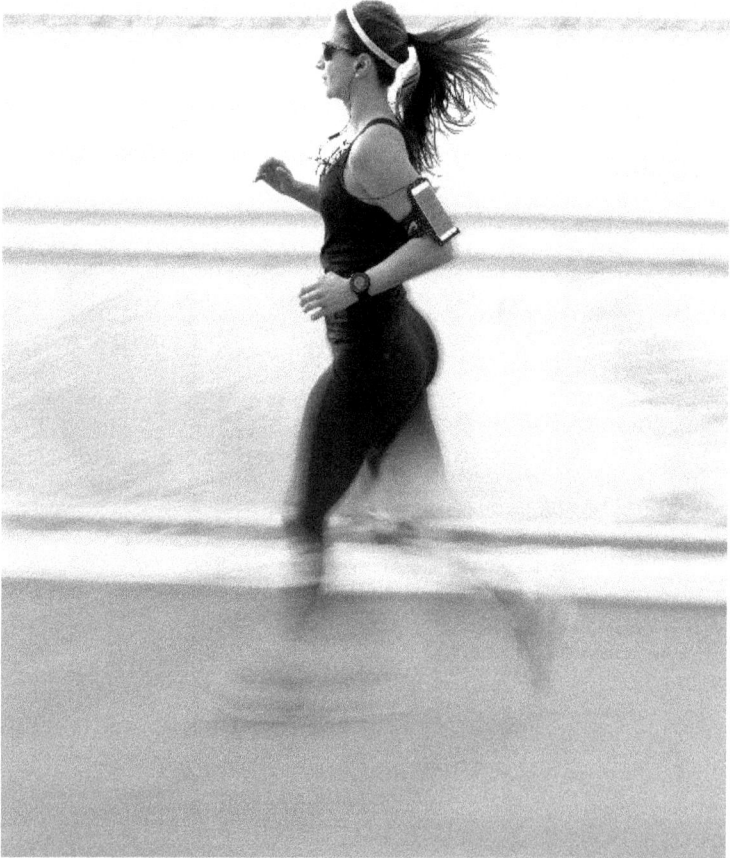

Finding Balance for Body and Mind

# Chapter 3

# Physical Activity and Fitness

## The Benefits of Regular Exercise

Regular exercise is an essential component of a healthy lifestyle, offering a multitude of benefits that extend beyond physical appearance. Engaging in consistent physical activity can significantly enhance one's overall well-being. It promotes cardiovascular health, strengthens muscles, and improves flexibility and balance.

By maintaining a regular exercise routine, individuals can reduce the risk of chronic illnesses such as heart disease, diabetes, and obesity. The physiological changes that occur during exercise, such as improved circulation and oxygen delivery, contribute to a stronger, more resilient body.

In addition to the physical benefits, regular exercise plays a crucial role in mental health. Engaging in physical activity releases endorphins, often referred to as "feel-good" hormones, which can lead to improved mood and reduced feelings of stress and anxiety. Regular workouts can help combat depression and increase overall emotional resilience.

Furthermore, exercise provides an opportunity for individuals to practice mindfulness, as physical activity often requires focus and presence, allowing the mind to detach from daily stressors and distractions.

Social benefits also arise from regular exercise. Participating in group activities, such as fitness classes or team sports, fosters connections with like-minded individuals, creating a supportive community. This social interaction can combat feelings of loneliness and isolation, contributing to a greater sense of belonging.

Building relationships through shared fitness goals not only enhances motivation but also encourages accountability, making it easier to stick to an exercise regimen.

Moreover, regular physical activity can lead to improved sleep quality. Individuals who engage in consistent exercise often experience deeper, more restorative sleep, which is essential for overall health. Quality sleep is vital for cognitive function, emotional regulation, and physical recovery.

By establishing a routine that incorporates exercise, individuals may find it easier to fall asleep and stay asleep, enhancing their daily performance and overall mood.

Finally, the benefits of regular exercise extend to personal development and self-esteem. Achieving fitness goals, whether they are small milestones or significant transformations, instills a sense of accomplishment and boosts confidence.

This newfound self-assurance can permeate other areas of life, encouraging individuals to pursue other healthy habits and goals. By prioritizing physical activity, individuals not only improve their health but also cultivate a positive mindset that contributes to a happier, more fulfilling life.

# Finding the Right Exercise for You

Finding the right exercise for you is crucial in your journey towards health and happiness. Exercise is not a one-size-fits-all approach; it varies significantly based on individual preferences, physical condition, and lifestyle. To begin this process, it's essential to consider what activities excite and motivate you. Engaging in exercises that bring joy can enhance adherence and make the pursuit of fitness feel less like a chore and more like a rewarding experience.

An important step in finding the right exercise is to assess your current fitness level and any physical limitations you may have. This self-assessment can help you identify which types of exercise might be suitable.

For instance, if you have joint issues, low-impact activities such as swimming, cycling, or yoga might be better choices compared to high-impact sports. Consulting with a healthcare professional or a personal trainer can provide tailored recommendations based on your specific needs and goals.

Exploring various forms of exercise can also be beneficial. Many people find joy in group classes, such as Zumba, Pilates, or martial arts, as they foster a sense of community and accountability. Others may prefer solo activities like running, hiking, or weightlifting, which allow for personal reflection and focus.

Experimenting with different workouts can help you discover what resonates with you, transforming exercise from a mundane obligation into an enjoyable part of your daily routine.

Considering your lifestyle and schedule is another vital aspect of choosing the right exercise. Busy professionals or parents may find it challenging to commit to lengthy workout sessions. In such cases, incorporating shorter, high-intensity workouts or utilizing bodyweight exercises that require minimal equipment can be effective.

The key is to create a routine that fits seamlessly into your life, making it easier to prioritize your health and well-being without feeling overwhelmed.

Lastly, remember that your exercise preferences may evolve over time. As you progress in your fitness journey or your circumstances change, it's essential to remain open to trying new activities. This adaptability can prevent boredom and keep your workouts fresh and exciting.

Ultimately, finding the right exercise for you is about creating a balanced approach that aligns with your personal interests, goals, and lifestyle, contributing positively to your overall health and happiness.

## Creating a Sustainable Fitness Routine

Creating a sustainable fitness routine involves more than simply adhering to a strict exercise schedule; it requires a holistic approach that aligns with individual lifestyles, preferences, and goals. To establish a routine that you can maintain over the long term, it is essential to begin by assessing your current physical condition, interests, and available resources. This self-assessment will help you identify the types of activities that resonate with you and the time you can realistically dedicate to fitness.

Understanding your motivations, whether they stem from health concerns, aesthetic goals, or stress relief, will also guide your choices and ensure that your routine remains engaging and fulfilling.

Incorporating a variety of exercises is crucial for both sustainability and overall fitness. While many people may gravitate towards popular activities like running or weightlifting, exploring different forms of exercise can prevent boredom and reduce the risk of injury. Consider mixing cardiovascular workouts, strength training, flexibility exercises, and recreational sports.

This diversity not only keeps the routine interesting but also addresses different aspects of physical health, enhancing endurance, strength, and mobility. Additionally, trying new activities such as yoga, swimming, or dance classes can introduce social elements that further motivate you to stay active.

# How To Be Healthy and Happy

Setting realistic goals plays a pivotal role in crafting a sustainable fitness routine. It is essential to establish specific, measurable, achievable, relevant, and time-bound (SMART) goals that align with your personal objectives. For instance, rather than aiming to "get fit," a more concrete goal might be to complete a 5K run within three months or to engage in strength training three times a week for four weeks.

These goals provide clear benchmarks for progress and encourage accountability. Celebrating small victories along the way can boost motivation and reinforce your commitment to the routine.

Consistency is key to maintaining any fitness regimen. To foster consistency, consider scheduling workouts as you would any other important appointment. Finding a time of day that works best for you, whether it's early morning, lunchtime, or after work, can help embed exercise into your daily routine.

Additionally, using tools such as fitness apps, journals, or community challenges can enhance accountability and encourage regular participation.

Establishing a support system, whether through workout buddies or online communities, can also provide encouragement and help you stay on track.

Lastly, listen to your body and prioritize recovery as part of your fitness routine. Sustainable fitness is not just about pushing your limits; it's also about respecting your physical needs and allowing time for rest and recovery. Incorporating rest days, ensuring adequate sleep, and maintaining a balanced diet are all integral components of a healthy routine.

By recognizing the importance of recovery, you can prevent burnout and injuries, ultimately leading to a more enjoyable and sustainable fitness experience. A well-rounded approach that includes listening to your body will help you find balance and contribute to your overall health and happiness.

# How To Be Healthy and Happy

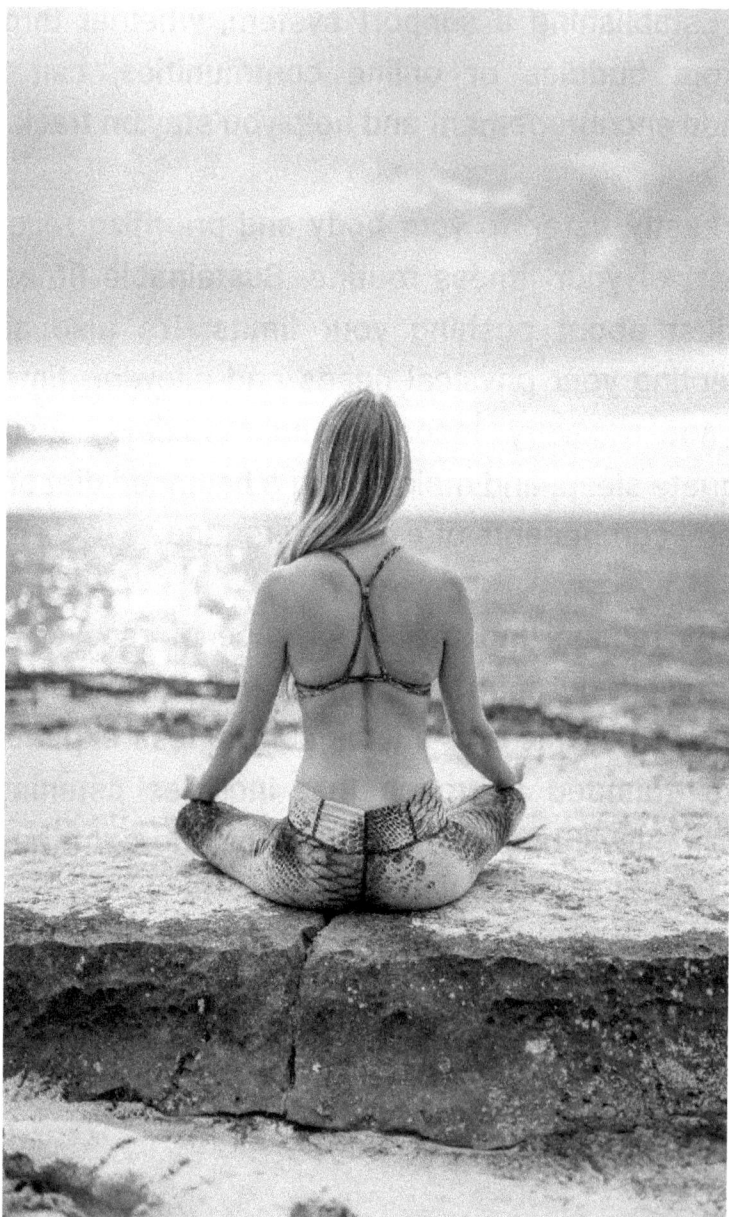

Finding Balance for Body and Mind

# Chapter 4

# Mental Wellness and Mindfulness

## The Role of Mental Health in Overall Wellbeing

Mental health plays a critical role in overall wellbeing, acting as the foundation on which physical health and emotional stability are built. When individuals prioritize their mental health, they often notice significant improvements in various aspects of their lives.

This includes enhanced relationships, better coping mechanisms, and an increased ability to manage stress. Understanding the interconnectedness of mental health with other components of wellbeing is essential for anyone seeking a balanced and fulfilling life.

The relationship between mental health and physical health is particularly noteworthy. Research has consistently shown that mental health disorders can lead to physical health issues, such as cardiovascular disease and weakened immune function.

Conversely, individuals who maintain good mental health often engage in healthier lifestyle choices, including regular exercise and balanced nutrition. These choices not only improve physical health but also contribute to a positive feedback loop that reinforces mental wellbeing, creating a cycle of health that benefits both the mind and body.

Emotional wellbeing is another facet deeply influenced by mental health. People who cultivate resilience and practice mindfulness tend to experience higher levels of happiness and satisfaction in life. They are better equipped to handle the inevitable stressors and challenges that arise, which can lead to a sense of empowerment. By implementing techniques such as meditation, journaling, or therapy, individuals can enhance their emotional intelligence, leading to improved relationships and a greater ability to empathize with others.

Social connections are also significantly impacted by mental health. Individuals who prioritize their mental wellbeing are generally more capable of forming and maintaining healthy relationships.

They communicate effectively, resolve conflicts constructively, and provide support to others. This social support network is vital for both mental and physical health, as it fosters a sense of belonging and reduces feelings of isolation. Engaging in community activities or maintaining friendships can serve as a protective factor against mental health challenges.

In conclusion, mental health is an integral component of overall wellbeing that cannot be overlooked. It influences physical health, emotional stability, and social interactions, all of which contribute to a holistic sense of happiness.

By recognizing the importance of mental health and actively seeking ways to improve it, individuals can enhance their quality of life. This journey towards better mental health is not only beneficial for oneself but also for the community, fostering a healthier and happier society.

## Introduction to Mindfulness Practices

Mindfulness practices have gained significant attention in recent years as a powerful tool for enhancing overall well-being. At its core, mindfulness involves cultivating a heightened awareness of the present moment, allowing individuals to observe their thoughts, feelings, and bodily sensations without judgment.

This practice encourages a deeper connection to oneself, fostering an environment in which individuals can experience life more fully. By incorporating mindfulness into daily routines, people may find that they can reduce stress, improve emotional regulation, and enhance their overall sense of happiness.

The origins of mindfulness can be traced back to ancient contemplative traditions, particularly in Buddhism. However, its principles have been adapted and integrated into modern psychological practices, making mindfulness accessible to a broader audience. Research has shown that mindfulness can have a profound impact on mental health, including reducing symptoms of anxiety and depression.

By focusing on the present moment, individuals can break free from the cycle of negative thinking that often contributes to emotional distress, paving the way for a healthier mindset.

Incorporating mindfulness into daily life can take many forms, including meditation, mindful breathing, and mindful eating. Each of these practices encourages individuals to slow down, reflect, and engage with their experiences fully.

For instance, meditation often involves sitting quietly and directing attention towards the breath or a particular thought, allowing distractions to come and go without attachment. Mindful eating encourages individuals to savor each bite, appreciating the flavors and textures of their food, which can lead to healthier eating habits and improved digestion.

Moreover, mindfulness can be practiced in various settings, making it adaptable to individual lifestyles. Whether during a busy workday, while commuting, or at home, there are countless opportunities to integrate mindfulness into everyday activities.

Simple techniques, such as taking a few deep breaths or pausing to notice one's surroundings, can significantly enhance one's awareness and appreciation for life. These practices not only promote relaxation but also create space for self-reflection and personal growth.

As individuals embark on their journey toward a healthier and happier life, embracing mindfulness practices can be a transformative step. By prioritizing present-moment awareness, individuals can cultivate resilience against stressors and develop a more profound sense of contentment.

The integration of mindfulness into daily routines is not just about achieving a temporary state of calm; it is about fostering a lasting shift in perspective that allows for a richer, more balanced life. In the chapters that follow, we will explore practical techniques and strategies to incorporate mindfulness into your lifestyle, empowering you to enhance both your physical and mental well-being.

## Techniques for Reducing Stress

Stress is a common experience that can significantly impact both physical and mental well-being. To manage stress effectively, individuals can employ various techniques that promote relaxation and foster a sense of calm. Understanding these techniques is crucial for anyone looking to enhance their overall health and happiness. By incorporating these methods into daily routines, individuals can reduce the negative effects of stress and cultivate a more balanced lifestyle.

One effective technique for reducing stress is mindfulness meditation. This practice involves focusing on the present moment while observing thoughts and feelings without judgment. By dedicating just a few minutes each day to mindfulness meditation, individuals can develop greater awareness of their stress triggers and learn to respond to them more calmly.

Research shows that regular mindfulness practice can lead to lower levels of anxiety and a more positive outlook on life, making it a valuable tool for anyone seeking to improve their mental health.

Another practical approach to stress management is physical exercise. Engaging in regular physical activity not only enhances physical fitness but also releases endorphins, which are natural mood lifters. Whether it's a brisk walk, yoga, or a more intense workout, exercise helps to alleviate stress by providing an outlet for pent-up energy and tension.

Furthermore, the rhythmic nature of many physical activities can induce a meditative state, allowing the mind to clear and refocus, which contributes to overall emotional well-being.

Breathing techniques are also essential for managing stress. Deep, controlled breathing can activate the body's relaxation response, counteracting the physiological effects of stress. Techniques such as diaphragmatic breathing, where one breathes deeply into the abdomen rather than shallowly into the chest, can help lower heart rate and blood pressure. Practicing these techniques for a few minutes throughout the day can provide immediate relief from stress and foster a greater sense of calm.

Finally, fostering social connections is a crucial aspect of stress reduction. Spending time with friends and loved ones can provide emotional support and a sense of belonging, both of which are important for mental health. Engaging in meaningful conversations and shared activities can help individuals feel more grounded and less isolated in their experiences.

Building a strong support network encourages individuals to express their feelings and seek help when needed, ultimately contributing to a healthier, happier lifestyle. Embracing these techniques can lead to significant improvements in one's ability to cope with stress and enhance overall well-being.

# How To Be Healthy and Happy

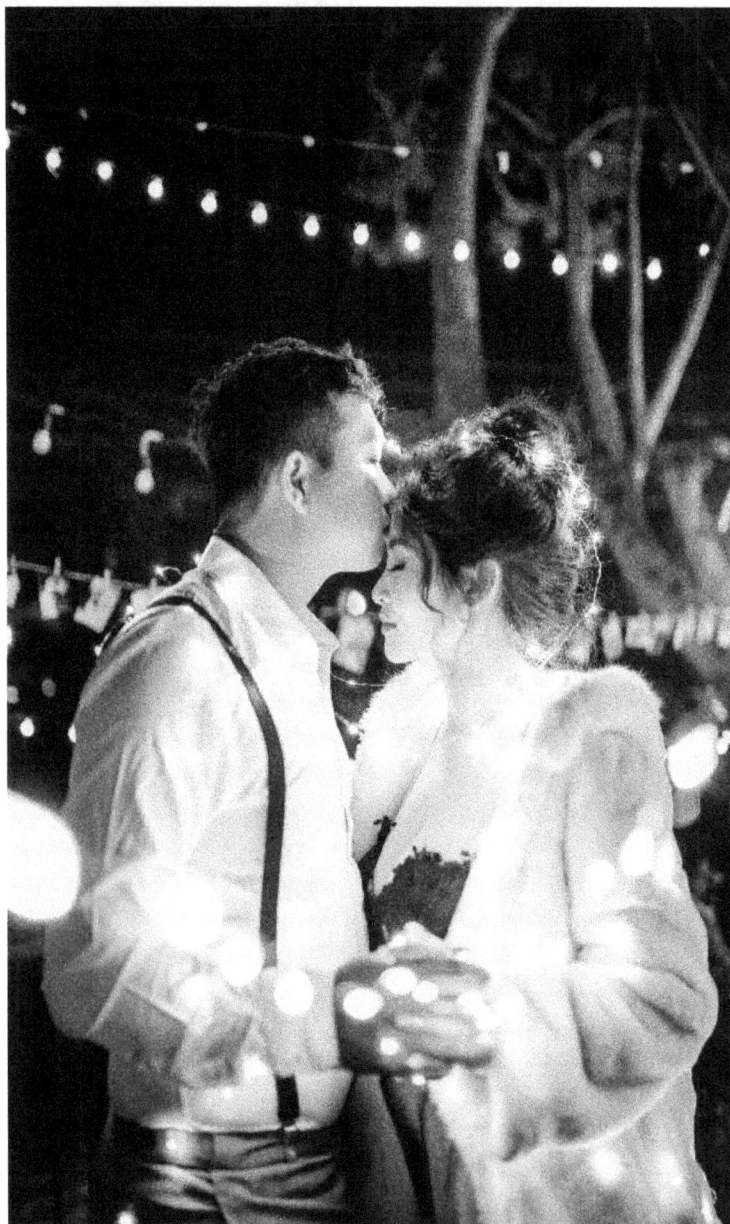

# Chapter 5

# Building Healthy Relationships

## The Impact of Relationships on Health

The impact of relationships on health is a crucial aspect of overall well-being that often goes overlooked. Numerous studies indicate that social connections can significantly influence both mental and physical health. Strong relationships provide emotional support, which can reduce stress and promote a sense of belonging.

Conversely, social isolation can lead to feelings of loneliness, anxiety, and depression, which in turn can have negative effects on one's physical health. Understanding the dynamics of these relationships is essential for anyone seeking to improve their overall health and happiness.

Healthy relationships can lead to better health outcomes. Positive interactions with friends, family, and loved ones contribute to lower blood pressure, improved immune function, and even longer life expectancy. The emotional support gleaned from these interactions helps individuals cope with stress more effectively, reducing the likelihood of chronic conditions such as heart disease or diabetes.

Furthermore, engaging in social activities can encourage healthier lifestyle choices, such as regular exercise and balanced eating, as individuals often motivate one another to maintain healthy habits.

Conversely, toxic relationships can detrimentally affect health. Relationships characterized by conflict, negativity, or lack of support can lead to chronic stress, which is known to cause various health issues, including cardiovascular problems and weakened immune responses. The emotional toll of such relationships can also contribute to mental health challenges, exacerbating conditions like anxiety and depression. Recognizing and addressing these unhealthy dynamics is essential for anyone looking to foster a healthier and happier life.

Building and maintaining healthy relationships requires intentional effort. Communication is key; openly discussing feelings, needs, and boundaries can strengthen bonds and foster mutual understanding.

Additionally, investing time in nurturing these relationships, whether through shared activities or simply being present, is vital. Practicing gratitude and expressing appreciation for loved ones can also enhance relationship satisfaction, promoting a positive feedback loop that benefits both parties' health.

Ultimately, the interplay between relationships and health underscores the importance of cultivating a supportive social network. Individuals concerned with their health and happiness should not only focus on physical well-being but also prioritize emotional and social health.

By fostering positive relationships and addressing those that are detrimental, individuals can significantly enhance their overall quality of life, leading to a more balanced and fulfilling existence.

## Effective Communication Skills

Effective communication skills are essential for fostering healthy relationships and promoting overall well-being. The ability to express oneself clearly and listen actively can significantly impact personal and professional interactions. Communication is not merely about exchanging words; it involves understanding emotions, intentions, and non-verbal cues. By honing these skills, individuals can enhance their connections with others, contributing to a more fulfilling and balanced life.

Active listening is a fundamental component of effective communication. It requires full attention to the speaker, allowing individuals to understand not only the words being spoken but also the underlying emotions.

Practicing active listening involves maintaining eye contact, nodding in acknowledgment, and refraining from interrupting. This skill encourages empathy and validation, making the speaker feel heard and respected. In turn, this can lead to deeper, more meaningful conversations and relationships that nurture mental and emotional health.

Clarity in expression is another vital aspect of effective communication. When individuals articulate their thoughts and feelings clearly, it minimizes misunderstandings and conflicts. Using simple language, being concise, and staying on topic are key strategies to enhance clarity. It is equally important to be mindful of the tone and body language used during interactions. A positive tone and open body language can convey warmth and approachability, making others more receptive to the message being delivered.

Moreover, providing and receiving constructive feedback is a crucial element of effective communication. Feedback should be specific, focusing on behaviors rather than personal attributes. When giving feedback, it is important to frame it positively, highlighting strengths before addressing areas for improvement.

Conversely, when receiving feedback, individuals should remain open-minded and view it as an opportunity for growth. This exchange fosters a culture of respect and continuous improvement, which is beneficial for personal development and interpersonal relationships.

Finally, practicing vulnerability can significantly enhance communication skills. Sharing personal thoughts and feelings, even in difficult situations, can build trust and intimacy in relationships. Vulnerability encourages authenticity, allowing individuals to connect on a deeper level. By embracing openness, people can create environments where honest dialogue flourishes, ultimately leading to greater emotional health and happiness. In summary, effective communication skills are indispensable for achieving a balanced and fulfilling life, providing the foundation for healthy relationships and emotional well-being.

## Setting Boundaries for Healthy Interactions

Setting boundaries is a crucial aspect of cultivating healthy interactions in both personal and professional relationships. It involves clearly defining what is acceptable behavior from others and what is not. Establishing these limits helps individuals protect their emotional and mental well-being while fostering respect and understanding in their interactions. Without clear boundaries, relationships can become strained, leading to feelings of resentment, anxiety, and even burnout.

One of the first steps in setting boundaries is self-awareness. Individuals must understand their own needs, values, and limits. This process often involves reflecting on past experiences and recognizing situations where personal boundaries were crossed. By identifying these moments, individuals can articulate what they need from their relationships moving forward. Practicing self-awareness not only aids in boundary setting but also enhances communication skills, making it easier to express needs and expectations to others.

Communication plays a vital role in establishing and maintaining boundaries. It is essential to convey limits clearly and assertively, without ambiguity. This includes expressing feelings and needs directly, using "I" statements to take ownership of one's emotions. For instance, instead of saying, "You always interrupt me," one might say, "I feel undervalued when I am interrupted during conversations." This approach promotes a non-confrontational dialogue and encourages the other party to understand and respect one's boundaries.

In addition to communication, consistency is key in boundary setting. Once boundaries are established, they must be upheld to ensure respect from others. Inconsistent enforcement can lead to confusion and may encourage others to disregard the established limits.

It is important to be prepared for resistance or pushback, particularly from those who may not be accustomed to the new boundaries. Remaining firm yet respectful in these situations reinforces the importance of the boundaries and demonstrates commitment to personal well-being.

Lastly, setting boundaries is not a one-time effort but an ongoing process that requires regular reflection and adjustment. As relationships evolve and circumstances change, individuals may find that their boundaries need to be reevaluated. Engaging in open conversations periodically can help ensure that boundaries remain relevant and respected. Embracing this dynamic approach not only enhances personal health and happiness but also contributes to more fulfilling and respectful interactions with others, ultimately leading to a more balanced life.

# How To Be Healthy and Happy

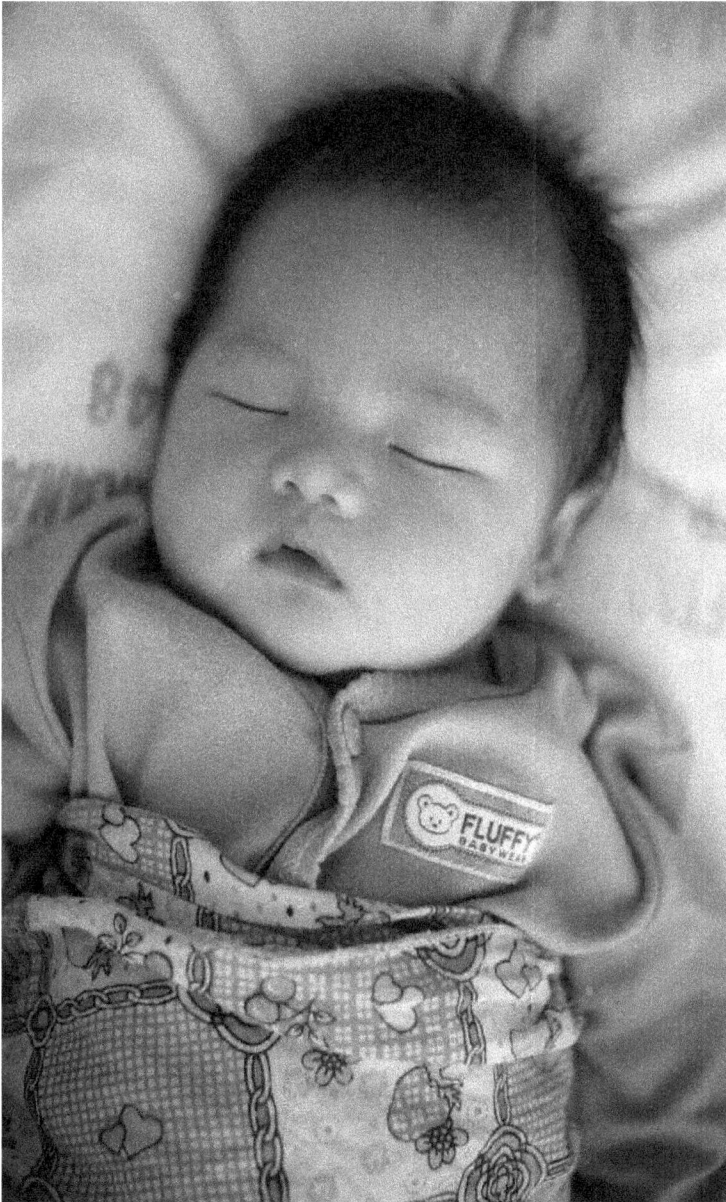

# Chapter 6

# Sleep and Recovery

## The Importance of Sleep for Health

Sleep is a fundamental aspect of overall health and well-being that is often overlooked in the pursuit of a balanced life. During sleep, the body undergoes critical restorative processes that are essential for physical and mental health. Adequate sleep allows for the replenishment of energy reserves, repair of tissues, and the regulation of hormones.

It is during these hours of rest that the brain consolidates memories, processes information, and clears out toxins. Understanding the significance of sleep can empower individuals to prioritize it as a vital component of their health regimen.

The relationship between sleep and mental health is profound. Studies have shown that insufficient sleep can lead to increased levels of stress, anxiety, and depression. When individuals do not get enough restorative sleep, their emotional regulation becomes compromised, leading to mood swings and irritability.

Additionally, chronic sleep deprivation can exacerbate existing mental health conditions and hinder recovery from emotional distress. Prioritizing sleep can therefore serve as a protective factor, enhancing resilience against mental health challenges and promoting a more stable emotional state.

Physical health is deeply intertwined with sleep quality and quantity. Research indicates that lack of sleep is linked to a higher risk of various medical conditions, including obesity, diabetes, cardiovascular disease, and weakened immune function. Sleep deprivation can disrupt metabolic processes, leading to weight gain and increased appetite. Furthermore, quality sleep supports a healthy immune response, enabling the body to fend off illness and recover more efficiently.

By recognizing the importance of sleep, individuals can take proactive steps to improve their overall health and reduce the likelihood of developing chronic illnesses.

Establishing healthy sleep habits is essential for maximizing the benefits of rest. Creating a consistent sleep schedule by going to bed and waking up at the same time each day can help regulate the body's internal clock. Additionally, creating a restful sleep environment—free of distractions like screens and excessive noise—can enhance sleep quality.

Engaging in relaxation techniques before bed, such as meditation or gentle stretching, can also prepare the mind and body for a restful night. By adopting these practices, individuals can cultivate an environment conducive to healthy sleep.

In conclusion, understanding the importance of sleep is crucial for anyone seeking to achieve a healthy and happy lifestyle. Adequate sleep not only supports physical health and emotional well-being but is also a foundational element of a balanced life.

By prioritizing sleep and implementing strategies to improve sleep hygiene, individuals can enhance their overall quality of life, increase their productivity, and foster a greater sense of happiness. Embracing the value of sleep as an integral part of health can lead to transformative changes in both body and mind.

## Sleep Hygiene Practices

Sleep hygiene practices are essential for maintaining optimal health and well-being. Quality sleep significantly impacts both physical and mental health, influencing mood, cognitive function, and overall vitality.

To cultivate good sleep hygiene, it is crucial to establish a consistent sleep schedule. This involves going to bed and waking up at the same time every day, even on weekends.

By regulating your body's internal clock, you can enhance the quality of your sleep and make it easier to fall asleep and wake up feeling refreshed.

Creating a restful sleep environment is another fundamental aspect of sleep hygiene. A dark, quiet, and cool room promotes better sleep. Consider using blackout curtains to block out light, earplugs or white noise machines to drown out disruptive sounds, and maintaining a temperature that feels comfortable for you. Additionally, investing in a comfortable mattress and pillows can make a significant difference in your ability to fall and stay asleep. Personalizing your sleep space can transform it into a sanctuary that encourages relaxation and rest.

Establishing a pre-sleep routine can also enhance sleep hygiene. Engaging in calming activities before bed, such as reading, taking a warm bath, or practicing mindfulness meditation, can signal to your body that it is time to wind down.

It is advisable to limit exposure to screens from phones, tablets, and computers at least an hour before bedtime, as the blue light emitted by these devices can interfere with the production of melatonin, the hormone responsible for regulating sleep. Instead, opt for activities that promote relaxation and prepare your mind for rest.

Diet and lifestyle choices play a vital role in sleep hygiene as well. Consuming heavy meals, caffeine, or alcohol close to bedtime can disrupt sleep patterns. It is wise to be mindful of what you eat and drink in the hours leading up to sleep.

Instead, consider light snacks if you're hungry, and aim to finish eating a few hours before bedtime. Regular physical activity can also improve sleep quality, but it is best to avoid vigorous exercise too close to bedtime, as it may have a stimulating effect.

Lastly, managing stress and anxiety is crucial for good sleep hygiene. Techniques such as deep breathing exercises, journaling, or talking to a trusted friend can help alleviate worries that may otherwise keep you awake. If sleep issues persist, it may be beneficial to consult a healthcare professional to identify underlying causes or receive tailored advice.

By implementing these sleep hygiene practices, you can create a foundation for healthier sleep habits, ultimately contributing to a happier and more balanced life.

# Understanding Recovery and Rest

Recovery and rest are essential components of a holistic approach to health and happiness. Understanding these concepts is crucial for anyone seeking balance in their lives. Recovery refers to the process of regaining strength and well-being after physical or mental exertion, while rest is the time taken to relax and rejuvenate the body and mind.

Both elements contribute significantly to overall health, as they allow the body to repair itself, and the mind to refresh, ultimately leading to improved performance in daily activities.

The importance of physical recovery cannot be overstated. Engaging in regular exercise is beneficial, but without adequate recovery, the body can suffer from fatigue and increased risk of injury.

Muscles need time to repair and grow stronger, which typically occurs during periods of rest. Incorporating rest days into a fitness routine is vital, as it allows the body to rebuild and adapt to the stresses placed upon it.

Additionally, practices such as stretching, foam rolling, and proper hydration contribute to recovery and enhance overall physical health.

Mental recovery is equally important, especially in today's fast-paced world. Chronic stress can lead to burnout and various mental health issues. Taking time for mental rest can involve activities that promote relaxation and mindfulness, such as meditation, reading, or spending time in nature.

These practices help to clear the mind and reduce anxiety, allowing individuals to return to their daily responsibilities with renewed focus and energy. Recognizing the signs of mental fatigue and taking proactive steps to address it is key to maintaining mental well-being.

Sleep plays a critical role in both physical and mental recovery. Quality sleep is essential for the body to heal and regenerate on a cellular level, while also facilitating cognitive functions such as memory and decision-making. Establishing a regular sleep schedule, creating a restful environment, and practicing good sleep hygiene can significantly enhance sleep quality.

By prioritizing restorative sleep, individuals can improve their overall health, mood, and productivity, leading to a more balanced and fulfilling life.

Incorporating recovery and rest into daily routines is essential for achieving a healthy and happy lifestyle. This involves recognizing the need for breaks and setting boundaries to ensure that both the body and mind receive the care they require.

By understanding the significance of recovery and rest, individuals can foster resilience against stress, enhance their physical capabilities, and ultimately cultivate a deeper sense of happiness and satisfaction in their lives. Embracing these concepts is not just about improving health; it's about nurturing a harmonious balance that supports overall well-being.

# How To Be Healthy and Happy

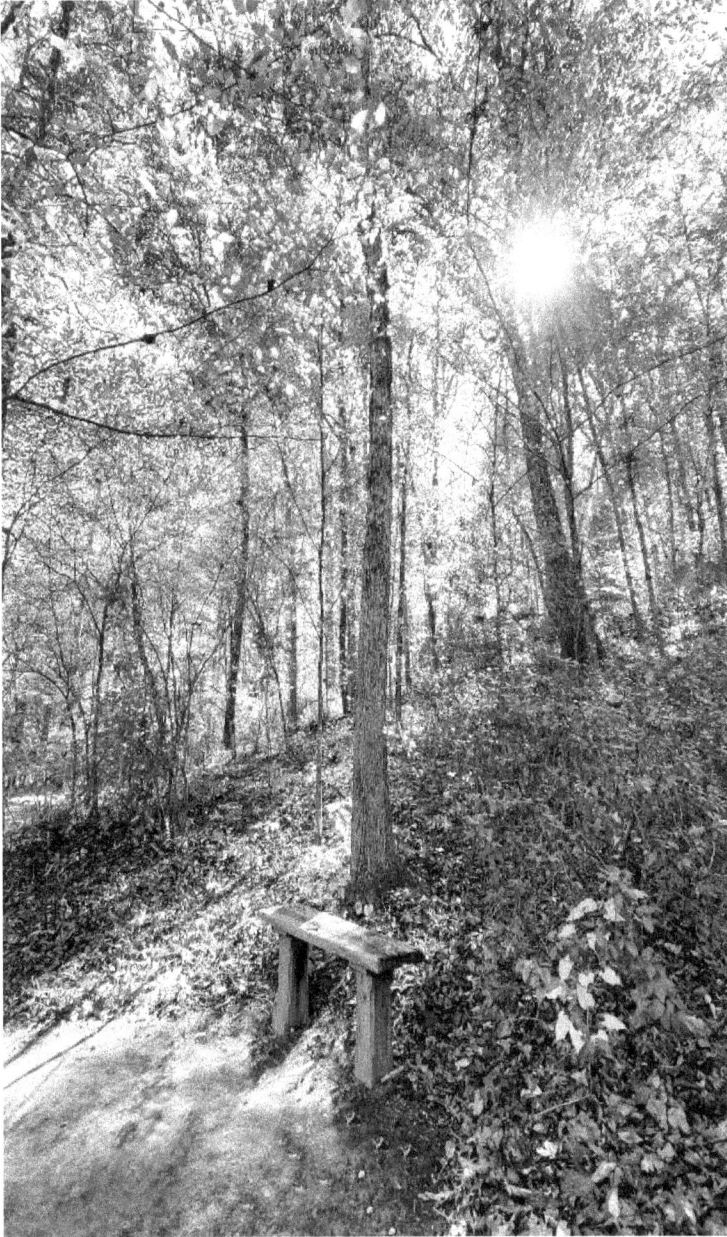

# Chapter 7

# Emotional Intelligence and Resilience

## What is Emotional Intelligence?

Emotional intelligence (EI) refers to the ability to recognize, understand, and manage our own emotions while also being able to recognize, understand, and influence the emotions of others. This concept encompasses several key components, including self-awareness, self-regulation, social awareness, and relationship management.

Individuals with high emotional intelligence are often more adept at navigating social complexities, managing stress, and making informed decisions that contribute to their overall well-being. By developing emotional intelligence, individuals can enhance their capacity for empathy and improve their interpersonal relationships, which are essential for achieving both health and happiness.

Self-awareness is the cornerstone of emotional intelligence. It involves being aware of one's emotions, strengths, weaknesses, and values. People with high self-awareness can recognize how their feelings affect their thoughts and behaviors, making them more capable of responding to situations thoughtfully rather than reacting impulsively.

This awareness can lead to healthier decision-making and a better understanding of how one's emotions influence interactions with others. Self-awareness is crucial for personal growth and can significantly impact overall happiness by fostering a deeper connection with oneself.

Self-regulation, another vital component of emotional intelligence, involves managing one's emotions in a constructive way. This means being able to control impulsive feelings and behaviors, which can lead to more thoughtful responses in challenging situations. Self-regulation allows individuals to maintain a sense of calm and stability, even in the face of stress or adversity. By mastering self-regulation, people can reduce anxiety and enhance their emotional resilience, contributing to a more balanced and fulfilling life.

Social awareness encompasses the ability to empathize with others and recognize their emotional cues. This skill is essential for building strong relationships and creating supportive environments, whether in personal or professional settings. Individuals who excel in social awareness can navigate social complexities and respond appropriately to the emotions of others.

This can lead to improved communication, collaboration, and conflict resolution, all of which are critical for fostering healthy relationships and a sense of community. Empathy, a key aspect of social awareness, also enriches one's life by deepening connections with others.

Relationship management involves using emotional intelligence to inspire, influence, and guide others effectively. This aspect of EI is about building healthy, meaningful relationships and maintaining them over time. Strong relationship management skills can lead to greater teamwork, improved leadership, and a more harmonious social environment.

In the pursuit of health and happiness, nurturing positive relationships is paramount, as they provide support, belonging, and joy. By cultivating emotional intelligence, individuals can enhance their ability to connect with others, leading to a more balanced and fulfilling life.

## Developing Resilience

Developing resilience is a crucial component in the pursuit of health and happiness. Resilience refers to the ability to bounce back from adversity, stress, and challenges, allowing individuals to maintain their well-being even in difficult circumstances. It involves a combination of mental, emotional, and behavioral flexibility, which enables a person to adapt to change and overcome obstacles.

By cultivating resilience, individuals can enhance their capacity to cope with life's ups and downs, ultimately leading to a more balanced and fulfilling life.

One of the foundational aspects of building resilience is fostering a positive mindset. This involves cultivating an attitude of optimism and reframing negative thoughts into more constructive ones. Practicing gratitude is a powerful tool in this regard. By focusing on what one is thankful for, individuals can shift their perspective from what is lacking or challenging to what is positive and enriching in their lives. Journaling about daily experiences and reflecting on positive moments can further reinforce this mindset, creating a buffer against stress and promoting overall mental well-being.

Another essential element in developing resilience is establishing a strong support system. Having a network of friends, family, or colleagues to lean on during tough times can provide encouragement, advice, and a sense of belonging.

It is important to nurture these relationships by maintaining open communication and being willing to both give and receive support. Engaging in community activities or support groups can also expand one's social circle, offering additional resources and shared experiences that strengthen resilience.

Self-care practices play a significant role in enhancing resilience as well. Regular physical exercise, a balanced diet, and adequate sleep are foundational to both physical and mental health. Engaging in mindfulness practices such as meditation, yoga, or deep breathing exercises can reduce stress and improve emotional regulation.

Additionally, setting aside time for hobbies and interests fosters joy and creativity, which can serve as a counterbalance to life's pressures. Prioritizing self-care not only contributes to resilience but also enhances overall happiness and satisfaction.

Finally, embracing a growth mindset is vital for developing resilience. This involves recognizing that challenges and failures are opportunities for learning and growth rather than insurmountable obstacles. By viewing setbacks as a natural part of the journey, individuals can approach difficulties with curiosity and determination rather than fear and avoidance. Setting realistic goals and celebrating progress, no matter how small, reinforces this mindset.

As individuals cultivate resilience through these practices, they lay the groundwork for a healthier and happier life, equipped to face whatever challenges may arise.

## Coping Strategies for Life Challenges

Coping strategies are essential tools for navigating life's challenges, as they help individuals maintain their mental and emotional well-being. Life inevitably presents obstacles, whether they are personal, professional, or health-related.

Understanding and implementing effective coping strategies can enable people to respond to stressors in a healthier manner, ultimately contributing to a more balanced and fulfilling life. These strategies can range from practical techniques to shifts in mindset, all aimed at fostering resilience and promoting happiness.

One effective coping strategy is the practice of mindfulness. Mindfulness involves being fully present in the moment, acknowledging one's thoughts and feelings without judgment. This practice can reduce anxiety and stress by helping individuals detach from overwhelming emotions.

Techniques such as deep breathing, meditation, or even simple awareness exercises can be incorporated into daily routines. Regular mindfulness practice encourages individuals to cultivate a sense of calm and clarity, which is particularly beneficial during challenging times.

Another valuable approach is the establishment of a support system. Building connections with friends, family, or support groups can provide emotional sustenance during difficult periods. Sharing experiences and feelings with others fosters a sense of belonging and reduces feelings of isolation. Moreover, seeking support from professionals, such as therapists or counselors, can offer new perspectives and coping techniques tailored to individual needs. Engaging with a community can create a network of encouragement, making challenges feel more manageable.

Physical activity is also a crucial component of coping with life challenges. Exercise has been shown to release endorphins, the body's natural mood lifters. Regular physical activity can alleviate symptoms of anxiety and depression while enhancing overall mood. Engaging in activities that one enjoys, whether it's walking, dancing, or practicing yoga, not only promotes physical health but also serves as a constructive outlet for stress. Incorporating movement into one's routine can significantly improve resilience and contribute to a happier, healthier life.

Finally, cultivating a positive mindset is a fundamental coping strategy for overcoming life's hurdles. This involves reframing negative thoughts and focusing on solutions rather than problems. Practices such as gratitude journaling can encourage individuals to recognize and appreciate the positive aspects of their lives, even during difficult times. Setting realistic goals and celebrating small achievements can also foster a sense of progress and motivation. By adopting a more optimistic outlook, individuals can better navigate challenges and enhance their overall sense of well-being.

In summary, coping strategies play a vital role in maintaining mental and emotional health during life's challenges. Mindfulness, building a support system, engaging in physical activity, and fostering a positive mindset are all effective approaches that can enhance resilience. By integrating these strategies into daily life, individuals can develop the tools necessary to face adversity with greater strength and ultimately cultivate a healthier, happier existence.

# How To Be Healthy and Happy

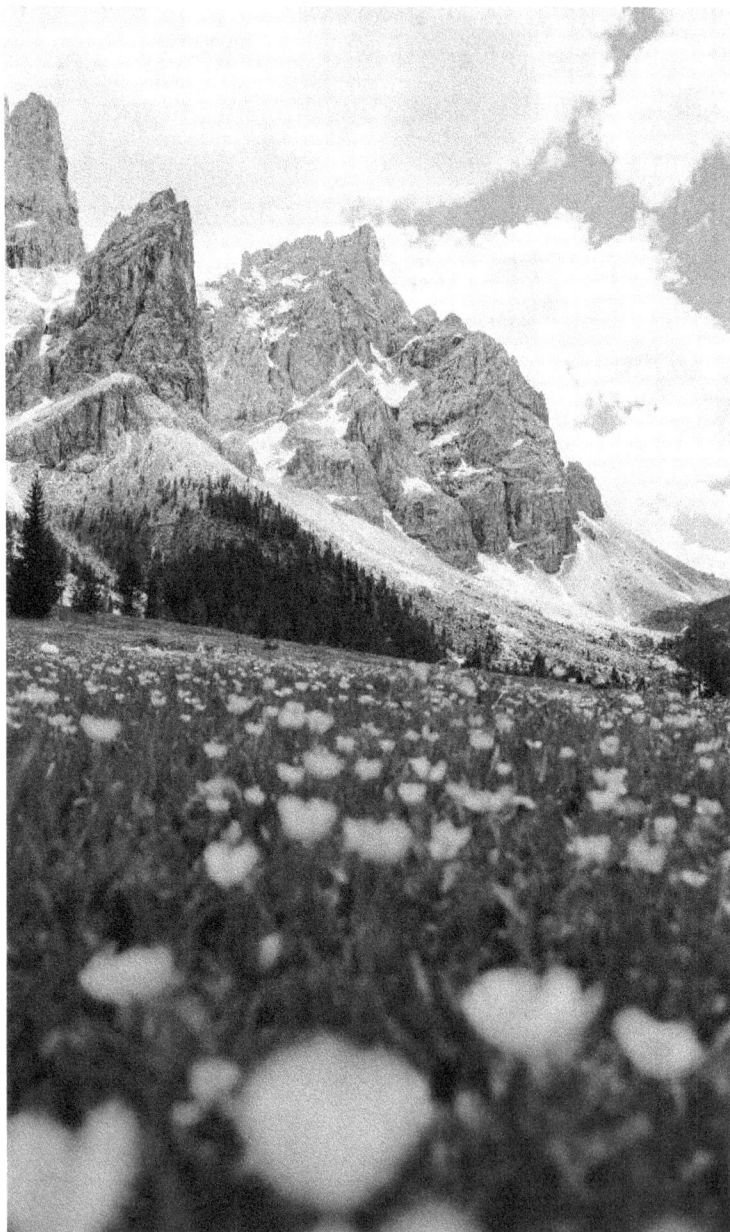

# Chapter 8

# Creating a Healthy Environment

## The Influence of Your Surroundings

The environment in which we live plays a crucial role in shaping our health and happiness. Our surroundings encompass not only the physical space we inhabit, such as our homes, neighborhoods, and workplaces, but also the social and cultural environments that influence our behaviors and attitudes.

Understanding the impact of these surroundings can help individuals make informed choices that promote well-being and foster a more balanced lifestyle.

Physical surroundings significantly affect our mental and physical health. For instance, living in a cluttered or disorganized space can lead to feelings of stress and anxiety, while a clean, well-organized environment can promote calmness and productivity. Natural elements, such as sunlight and greenery, have been shown to enhance mood and reduce stress levels.

Therefore, creating a living space that incorporates these elements can contribute to improved overall well-being. Additionally, accessibility to parks, recreational areas, and safe walking paths encourages physical activity, which is vital for both physical health and mental clarity.

Social environments are equally influential. The relationships we cultivate with family, friends, and colleagues can greatly impact our emotional state. Positive social interactions provide support, encouragement, and a sense of belonging, all of which are essential for happiness. Conversely, toxic relationships can lead to stress and unhappiness.

It is important to evaluate the quality of the relationships in one's life and to seek connections with individuals who uplift and inspire. Building a supportive community can lead to improved mental health outcomes and a greater sense of fulfillment.

Cultural influences also shape our health behaviors and perceptions. Societal norms can dictate what is considered healthy or acceptable, influencing our choices around diet, exercise, and self-care. Understanding these cultural factors allows individuals to critically assess their behaviors and make changes that align with their personal values and health goals. Embracing a culture of wellness—one that prioritizes healthy eating, regular physical activity, and mental well-being—can lead to positive changes and a more balanced life.

In conclusion, recognizing the profound influence of our surroundings on our health and happiness is essential for anyone seeking to improve their overall well-being. By being mindful of the physical, social, and cultural environments we inhabit, we can make deliberate choices that foster a healthier and happier life.

Creating a supportive, positive environment, both physically and socially, can lead to enhanced happiness and a greater sense of balance in body and mind.

## Decluttering and Organizing for Peace

Decluttering and organizing your living space can significantly contribute to your mental well-being. A cluttered environment often leads to a cluttered mind, creating stress and anxiety that can hinder your ability to focus and find peace.

By removing unnecessary items and organizing your surroundings, you create a calming atmosphere that encourages relaxation and clarity. This process not only enhances your physical space but also positively impacts your emotional state, making it easier to cultivate happiness and health.

Begin the decluttering process by assessing each area of your home. Start small, perhaps with a single drawer or a corner of a room. This manageable approach prevents feelings of overwhelm and allows you to see progress quickly.

As you sort through your belongings, ask yourself whether each item serves a purpose or brings you joy. Items that no longer fit into your life can be donated or recycled, enabling you to create space for things that truly matter. This act of letting go can be liberating and can foster a sense of accomplishment.

Once you have decluttered, organizing your space becomes the next vital step. Establish a system that works for you, whether it be by category, frequency of use, or location. Use storage solutions that maximize space, such as bins, shelves, and dividers, to keep items easily accessible yet out of sight.

An organized space not only looks appealing but also promotes productivity and efficiency, allowing you to focus on tasks without distraction. When everything has its place, the chances of chaos returning diminish, supporting a more serene environment.

Incorporating regular maintenance into your decluttering and organizing routine is essential for long-term peace. Schedule periodic check-ins to reassess your belongings and ensure that your space remains clutter-free.

This can be a monthly or seasonal activity, allowing you to adapt to any changes in your lifestyle or priorities. By making decluttering a habit, you reinforce a sense of control and mindfulness in your life, further contributing to your overall happiness and health.

Finally, consider the emotional and psychological aspects of decluttering and organizing. The process often brings up feelings of nostalgia, guilt, or attachment to items that may no longer serve you. Acknowledge these emotions and give yourself permission to feel them, but also remind yourself of the benefits of maintaining an organized space.

The clarity gained from a tidy environment can lead to improved mental health, reduced stress levels, and a greater sense of well-being. Ultimately, decluttering and organizing is not just about physical space; it is about creating a sanctuary that nurtures your body and mind, paving the way for a healthier, happier life.

## Incorporating Nature into Daily Life

Incorporating nature into daily life can significantly enhance one's overall health and happiness. One of the simplest ways to do this is by spending time outdoors. Engaging with natural environments—be it a park, a beach, or a forest—provides numerous physical and mental health benefits. Studies have shown that spending time in nature can reduce stress, improve mood, and enhance cognitive function.

By making a conscious effort to step outside, even for short periods, individuals can reap the rewards of fresh air and natural light, which are vital for both physical and psychological well-being.

Another effective method of integrating nature into daily routines is through gardening. Whether tending to a small indoor plant or cultivating a large garden, the act of nurturing plants can be incredibly fulfilling. Gardening not only promotes physical activity but also encourages mindfulness, as it requires focus and attention to detail.

The process of planting, watering, and watching plants grow fosters a connection to the earth, providing a sense of accomplishment and purpose. Moreover, the fresh produce harvested from a garden can contribute to a healthier diet, further enhancing overall well-being.

Incorporating nature into daily life can also be achieved through mindful practices such as nature walks or outdoor meditation. Taking a walk in natural settings allows individuals to connect with their surroundings, observe the beauty of the environment, and experience the calming effects of nature. Mindful walking encourages awareness of one's thoughts and feelings, promoting mental clarity and emotional resilience.

Similarly, practicing meditation outdoors can deepen the experience by harnessing the sights and sounds of nature to enhance focus and relaxation. By creating a regular routine that includes these activities, individuals can cultivate a greater sense of peace and balance in their lives.

Another approach to fostering a connection with nature is through sustainable living practices. Making conscious choices, such as reducing waste, using eco-friendly products, and supporting local wildlife, can create a sense of responsibility and stewardship toward the environment.

Engaging in activities like recycling, composting, or participating in community clean-up events not only benefits the planet but also fosters a sense of community and belonging.

This connection to a larger purpose can contribute to feelings of happiness and fulfillment, reinforcing the idea that individual actions can make a positive impact on both personal health and the health of the planet.

Finally, technology can be harnessed to facilitate a connection with nature. Many apps and online resources provide information on local parks, trails, and natural reserves, making it easier for individuals to discover outdoor spaces nearby.

Virtual reality experiences also offer an innovative way to explore natural environments from the comfort of home, providing a brief escape that can still impart feelings of tranquility. By finding creative ways to incorporate nature into daily life, individuals can enhance their health and happiness, leading to a more balanced and fulfilling existence.

# How To Be Healthy and Happy

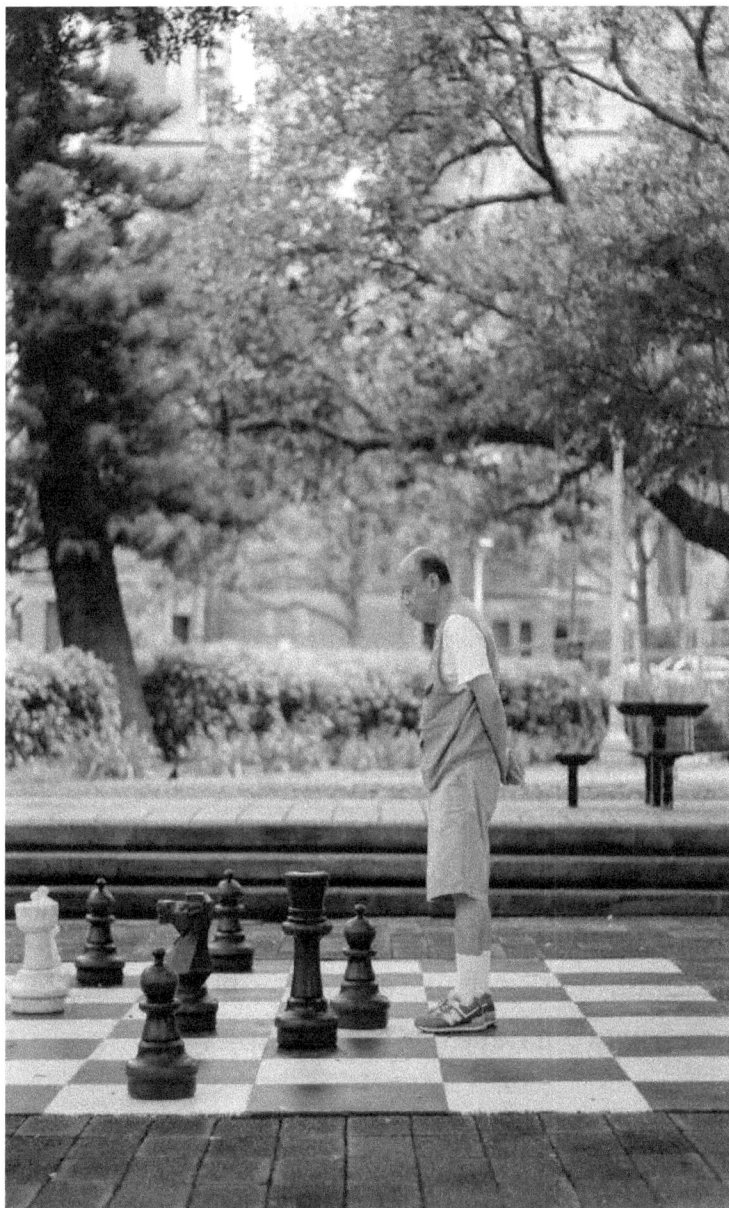

# Chapter 9

# Setting Goals for Health and Happiness

## The Importance of Goal Setting

Goal setting is a fundamental aspect of personal development that plays a crucial role in achieving health and happiness. By establishing clear and achievable goals, individuals can create a structured pathway toward their desired outcomes.

This process not only provides direction but also enhances motivation, making it easier to pursue lifestyle changes that contribute to overall well-being. Whether the goals are related to physical health, mental wellness, or overall life satisfaction, having a clear focus can significantly impact an individual's journey toward a healthier and happier life.

One of the primary benefits of goal setting is the ability to measure progress. When individuals set specific, measurable, attainable, relevant, and time-bound (SMART) goals, they can track their achievements more effectively. This tracking fosters a sense of accomplishment, which can be immensely motivating.

For instance, someone aiming to improve their fitness level might set a goal to run a certain distance within a specific timeframe. As they work toward this goal, every step of progress reinforces their commitment to their health journey, making it easier to maintain healthy habits over time.

Moreover, goal setting helps individuals to prioritize their efforts. In a world filled with distractions, it can be challenging to determine where to focus one's energy. By clearly defining goals, individuals can allocate their time and resources more effectively. This prioritization is particularly important in maintaining a healthy lifestyle, as it allows for the integration of nutritious eating, regular exercise, and mental health practices into daily routines.

When goals are prioritized, it becomes easier to say no to activities or habits that do not align with one's objectives, ultimately leading to a more balanced and fulfilling life.

Additionally, setting goals can enhance mental resilience. The journey toward achieving goals often involves overcoming obstacles and setbacks. By engaging in this process, individuals develop problem-solving skills and resilience, which are essential for maintaining mental health.

Each challenge faced and overcome reinforces the belief in one's ability to achieve, fostering a positive mindset. This mental fortitude not only contributes to personal growth but also aids in managing stress and anxiety, making it easier to navigate life's ups and downs.

Finally, the act of setting and pursuing goals can create a sense of purpose. Having clear objectives gives individuals something to strive for, which is vital for overall happiness.

This sense of purpose can enhance life satisfaction, as individuals feel more in control of their lives and more connected to their aspirations. In this way, goal setting is not just about achieving specific outcomes; it is a holistic practice that nurtures both the body and mind. By embracing this practice, individuals can pave the way toward a healthier, happier existence, ultimately finding the balance they seek.

## SMART Goals for Wellness

SMART goals are an effective framework for achieving wellness, as they provide a clear structure for setting and reaching health-related objectives. SMART is an acronym that stands for Specific, Measurable, Achievable, Relevant, and Time-bound. This method encourages individuals to break down their wellness aspirations into manageable components, making it easier to track progress and stay motivated.

By applying the SMART criteria, individuals can create actionable goals that align with their desire to cultivate a healthier and happier lifestyle.

Specificity is crucial when defining wellness goals. Instead of stating a vague intention such as "I want to be healthier," a specific goal could be "I will exercise for 30 minutes five times a week." This clarity helps in identifying precisely what needs to be done and removes ambiguity from the goal-setting process.

By honing in on particular areas, such as physical fitness, nutrition, or mental well-being, individuals can tailor their efforts to address specific aspects of their health.

Measurable goals allow individuals to track their progress and celebrate achievements along the way. For instance, instead of simply aiming to "eat better," a measurable goal could be "I will include at least two servings of vegetables in my meals each day."

This quantifiable approach enables individuals to see improvement over time, fostering a sense of accomplishment and reinforcing positive behaviors. Regularly monitoring these metrics helps maintain motivation and can also provide insights into what strategies are most effective.

Achievability is essential in goal-setting, as unrealistic expectations can lead to frustration and discouragement. Setting attainable goals involves considering current capabilities and resources. For example, someone new to exercise might aim for three 20-minute workouts per week rather than jumping straight into a rigorous routine.

By ensuring that goals are realistic, individuals are more likely to stick with their plans and gradually build confidence in their abilities, paving the way for more challenging objectives in the future.

Lastly, relevance and time-bound elements are vital in fostering a sense of purpose and urgency. Goals should align with personal values and overall life objectives, ensuring that the pursuit of wellness feels meaningful. Additionally, establishing a clear deadline, such as "I will achieve this goal within three months," creates a sense of urgency that can drive commitment. By integrating these SMART principles into their wellness journey, individuals can cultivate a balanced approach to health that not only enhances their physical well-being but also contributes to their overall happiness.

## Tracking Progress and Adjusting Goals

Tracking progress is essential for anyone seeking to maintain a healthy and happy lifestyle. It provides tangible evidence of what is working and highlights areas that may need adjustment. By regularly assessing both physical and mental health goals, individuals can stay motivated and focused on their journey.

This process not only fosters accountability but also empowers people to celebrate their achievements, no matter how small. Keeping a journal or using apps to monitor daily habits, such as exercise, nutrition, and emotional well-being, can serve as useful tools in this endeavor.

Establishing clear, measurable goals is the first step in tracking progress effectively. Goals should be specific, achievable, and time-bound to provide a clear roadmap. For instance, instead of stating a desire to "exercise more," a more effective goal would be to "walk for 30 minutes five days a week."

This clarity enables individuals to easily evaluate their efforts and successes. Additionally, breaking larger goals into smaller milestones can make the journey feel less overwhelming and more attainable, allowing for regular reassessment and celebration of progress.

Regularly reviewing progress allows for necessary adjustments to be made. Life is dynamic, and what works at one stage may not be effective later on. For example, if someone finds that their initial exercise routine is becoming monotonous or less effective, it may be time to introduce variety, such as trying new classes or outdoor activities.

Adjusting goals in response to progress not only keeps the journey engaging but also ensures that the pursuit of health and happiness remains aligned with one's evolving needs and circumstances.

In addition to physical measures, tracking emotional and mental health is equally important. This can involve reflecting on mood changes, stress levels, and overall satisfaction with life. Tools such as mood tracking apps or mindfulness practices can provide insight into emotional patterns and triggers.

By understanding these aspects, individuals can adjust their goals to prioritize mental well-being, whether that means incorporating stress-relief techniques or seeking professional support when needed. Recognizing that mental health is a crucial component of overall health is vital for achieving balance.

Ultimately, the journey toward health and happiness is ongoing and requires flexibility. It is essential to recognize that setbacks are a natural part of the process. When progress stalls or challenges arise, it is crucial to reassess both goals and methods, rather than seeing these moments as failures.

Embracing a mindset of growth and resilience can transform obstacles into opportunities for learning and development. By continually tracking progress and being willing to adjust goals, individuals can cultivate a sustainable path to a fulfilling and balanced life.

# How To Be Healthy and Happy

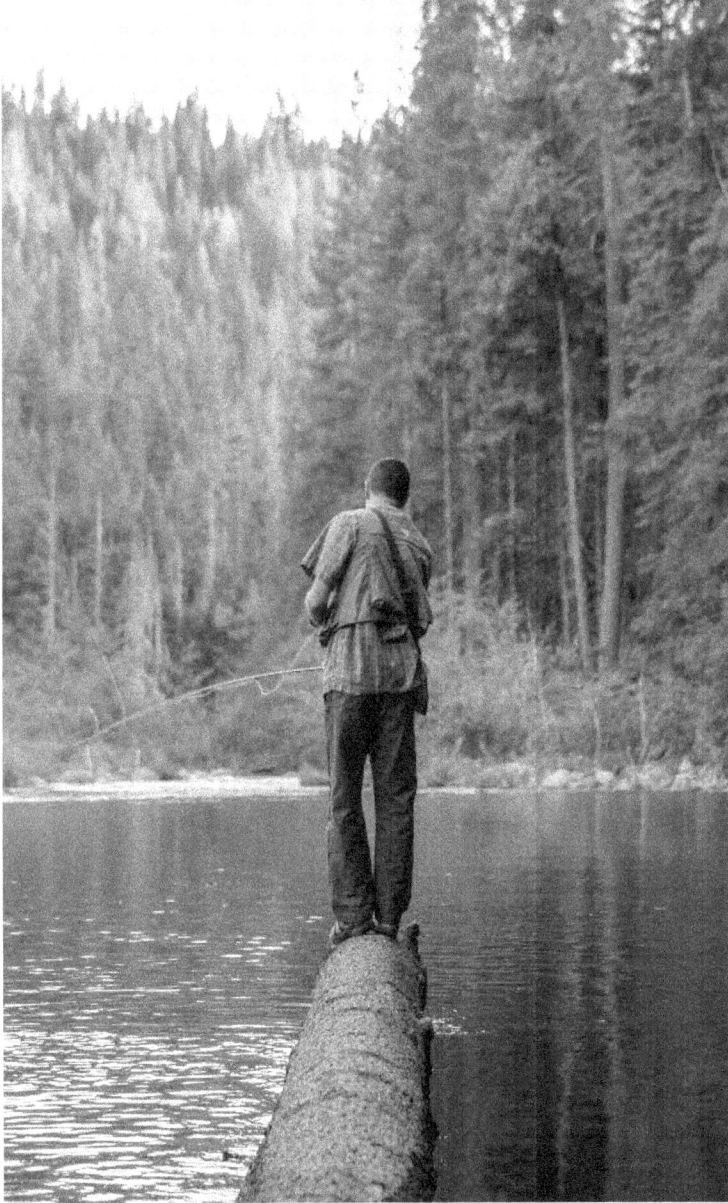

# Chapter 10

# Maintaining Balance in Daily Life

## Time Management for Health

Time management is a crucial skill for anyone seeking to improve their health and overall happiness. In a world filled with distractions and endless commitments, effectively managing time allows individuals to prioritize their well-being.

Allocating specific times for exercise, meal preparation, and relaxation can lead to healthier lifestyle choices. By creating a structured schedule, individuals can ensure they dedicate ample time to physical activity, nutritious eating, and mental wellness, which are all essential components of a balanced life.

One of the first steps in effective time management for health is setting clear goals. Goals should be specific, measurable, attainable, relevant, and time-bound (SMART). For example, instead of stating a vague intention to "exercise more," one might set a goal to "jog for 30 minutes three times a week." This clarity not only provides direction but also helps in tracking progress. By breaking down larger health objectives into smaller, actionable steps, individuals can maintain motivation and see tangible results over time.

Incorporating health-focused activities into a daily routine requires planning and prioritization. Identifying peak energy times throughout the day can assist in scheduling workouts or meal preparation when one is most likely to engage fully.

For instance, if a person feels more energized in the morning, they might choose to exercise first thing after waking up. Similarly, setting aside time in the evening to prepare healthy meals for the week can help mitigate the temptation of unhealthy fast food choices during busy days.

Time management also involves learning to say no to activities that do not align with health goals. This can be particularly challenging in a culture that often celebrates busyness. However, prioritizing personal health means recognizing that not every invitation or obligation must be accepted.

By being selective about commitments, individuals can free up time for activities that nurture both physical and mental health, such as yoga, meditation, or simply enjoying a quiet evening with a good book.

Finally, it is essential to build flexibility into time management strategies. Life can be unpredictable, and sticking rigidly to a plan may lead to frustration. Instead, adopting a mindset that allows for adjustments can help maintain balance. If a workout is missed or a meal is not prepped as planned, it is important to approach the situation without guilt.

By treating these challenges as opportunities for learning and adaptation, individuals can cultivate resilience, ultimately enhancing their journey toward a healthier and happier life.

## Finding Joy in Daily Activities

Finding joy in daily activities is essential for cultivating a healthy and happy life. Often, individuals overlook the small moments that can bring immense satisfaction and pleasure. Embracing these everyday experiences can significantly enhance one's overall well-being. It is vital to recognize that joy can be found not only in significant milestones but also in the mundane tasks of daily life. By shifting focus and appreciating these moments, people can transform their routines into sources of happiness.

One effective way to find joy in daily activities is through mindfulness. Practicing mindfulness involves being present and fully engaged in the moment, which allows individuals to savor their experiences.

Whether it's enjoying the aroma of a morning coffee, taking a leisurely stroll, or engaging in a conversation with a loved one, mindfulness helps individuals reconnect with their senses and appreciate the beauty of ordinary moments. This practice not only enhances emotional well-being but also reduces stress, leading to a healthier mindset.

Another strategy for discovering joy is to incorporate activities that align with personal interests and passions into daily routines. When individuals engage in tasks that resonate with them, they are more likely to experience satisfaction and fulfillment. For instance, someone who loves gardening may find joy in tending to their plants, while another person may derive happiness from cooking or painting. Finding ways to integrate these passions into everyday life can elevate a person's mood and create a sense of purpose.

Additionally, establishing a routine that includes moments of gratitude can significantly enhance one's ability to find joy. Taking time each day to reflect on positive experiences or express appreciation for simple pleasures can shift an individual's perspective.

This practice not only fosters a positive mindset but also encourages a greater awareness of the good things in life, making it easier to find joy in daily activities. Keeping a gratitude journal or sharing moments of thankfulness with friends and family can amplify this effect.

Finally, social connections play a crucial role in finding joy in daily activities. Engaging with others, whether through conversation, shared meals, or group activities, can enhance the enjoyment of everyday tasks. Building strong relationships fosters a sense of belonging and support, making routine activities more enjoyable.

By prioritizing social interactions, individuals can create opportunities for laughter, connection, and shared experiences, all of which contribute to a happier and healthier lifestyle.

## Strategies for Long-term Balance

Achieving long-term balance in life requires a multifaceted approach that encompasses physical health, mental well-being, and emotional stability. One effective strategy is to establish a consistent routine that promotes healthy habits. This includes setting specific times for meals, exercise, and relaxation.

By creating a structured daily schedule, individuals can ensure that they allocate time for self-care activities, which can significantly enhance overall well-being. A routine also helps reduce decision fatigue, allowing individuals to focus on maintaining their health and happiness without becoming overwhelmed.

Another vital strategy for long-term balance is prioritizing nutrition. A balanced diet rich in whole foods, such as fruits, vegetables, whole grains, lean proteins, and healthy fats, can have a profound impact on both physical and mental health. Individuals should aim to limit processed foods and added sugars, which can lead to energy crashes and mood swings.

Meal planning can be a useful tool in achieving this goal, as it allows individuals to prepare healthy meals in advance and make informed choices about their dietary habits. Staying hydrated is also essential, as proper hydration supports cognitive function and overall vitality.

Physical activity is another cornerstone of a balanced lifestyle. Regular exercise not only helps maintain a healthy weight but also boosts mood and reduces stress. Finding an enjoyable form of physical activity is crucial, whether it be dancing, hiking, swimming, or yoga. Incorporating movement into daily routines can also be beneficial, such as taking short breaks to stretch or walk. Setting realistic fitness goals can help individuals stay motivated and committed to their exercise routines, ultimately contributing to a sense of achievement and well-being.

Mental health is equally important in the pursuit of balance. Incorporating mindfulness practices, such as meditation or deep-breathing exercises, can greatly enhance emotional resilience and promote a positive mindset.

Engaging in activities that foster creativity and self-expression, such as painting, writing, or playing music, can also play a significant role in mental wellness. Additionally, maintaining social connections with friends and family provides emotional support and a sense of belonging, which are essential for long-term happiness.

Lastly, cultivating a positive outlook and practicing gratitude can significantly influence one's overall happiness. Keeping a gratitude journal, where individuals regularly write down things they are thankful for, can shift focus away from negativity and enhance appreciation for the present moment. This practice encourages individuals to recognize the positive aspects of their lives, even during challenging times.

By integrating these strategies into daily life, individuals can create a sustainable framework for achieving long-term balance, ultimately leading to a healthier and happier existence.

# Author Notes & Acknowledgments

First and foremost, I would like to express my deepest gratitude to the people who inspired and supported me throughout the journey of writing this book. This project would not have been possible without their unwavering belief in me and their invaluable contributions.

To my wife, thank you for your constant encouragement and understanding. Your love and support have been my anchor during the challenging times of researching and writing this book. Your belief in my ability to make a difference in people's lives has been my driving force.

I would also like to disclose that this book contains some renewed artificial intelligence-generated content. I really appreciate very recent technological innovation by outstanding scientists and of course our reader's understanding.

Lastly, I want to express my deepest gratitude to the readers of this book. I sincerely hope the strategies and methods outlined within these pages will provide you with the knowledge and tools needed to truly make your life much better. Your commitment to seeking any good solutions and willingness to explore multiple methods is commendable.

# Author Bio

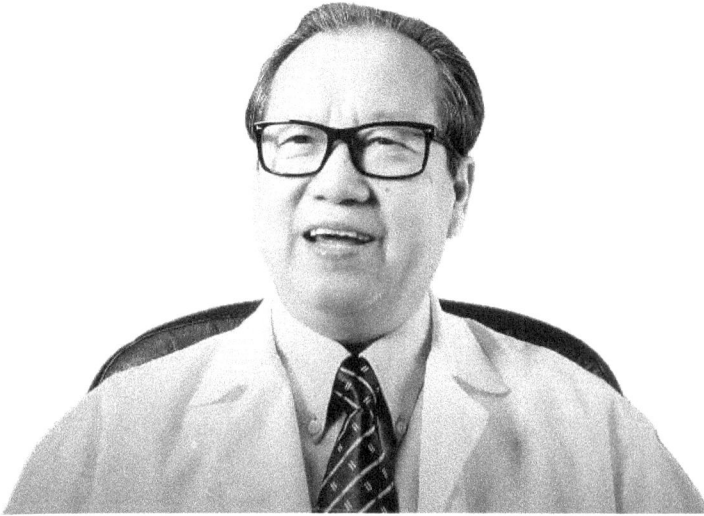

Johnson Wu earned his MD in 1982. With over 40 years of clinical experience, he has worked in hospitals in Zhejiang and Shanghai, China, as well as the Royal Marsden Hospital (part of Imperial College) in London, UK. Upon the recommendation of Sir Aaron Klug, the president of The Royal Society and a Nobel Prize winner in Chemistry, Dr. Wu was honorably awarded a British Royal Society Fellowship. He has published over 100 medical books in many countries and currently practices medicine in Canada.

www.ingramcontent.com/pod-product-compliance
Lightning Source LLC
Chambersburg PA
CBHW060250030426
42335CB00014B/1643